<u>Weight Training for Old Guys</u>

A Practical Guide for the Over-Fifty Crowd

(And Good Advice for the Rest of Us!)

Timothy Caso

Sports Performance Coach

Weight Training for Old Guys supports the **Wounded Warrior Project (WWP)**. Ten-percent of the proceeds from this book are donated to the **WWP**.

Published by BookLocker.com, Inc., St. Petersburg, Florida.

Printed on acid-free paper.

BookLocker.com, Inc.
2016

First Edition

DISCLAIMER

This book details the author's personal experiences with and opinions about physical fitness and weight training. The author is not a licensed medical practitioner.

The author and publisher are providing this book and its contents on an "as is" basis and make no representations or warranties of any kind with respect to this book or its contents. The author and publisher disclaim all such representations and warranties, including for example warranties of merchantability and fitness advice for a particular purpose. In addition, the author and publisher do not represent or warrant that the information accessible via this book is accurate, complete or current.

The statements made about products and services have not been evaluated by the U.S. government. Please consult with your own legal or accounting professional regarding the suggestions and recommendations made in this book.

Except as specifically stated in this book, neither the author or publisher, nor any authors, contributors, or other representatives will be liable for damages arising out of or in connection with the use of this book. This is a comprehensive limitation of liability that applies to all damages of any kind, including (without limitation) compensatory; direct, indirect or consequential damages; loss of data, income or profit; loss of or damage to property and claims of third parties.

You understand that this book is not intended as a substitute for consultation with a licensed medical, legal or accounting professional. Before you begin any change your lifestyle in any way, you will consult a licensed professional to ensure that you are doing what's best for your situation.

This book provides content related to physical fitness topics. As such, use of this book implies your acceptance of this disclaimer.

Table Of Contents

Chapter I
Introduction: Get Real

Let's face it: we're old. Fifty is not the new thirty (we wish). Fifty is fifty. If *spry* is the last word you would use to describe yourself when you get up in the morning or off the couch after the game, then you've come to the right place, and this book is for you! Like it or not, we are not part of the supple-jointed generation anymore! As they say, that ship has sailed. Stiffness, soreness, limps we didn't know we had— yes, we fifty-and-over folk are staring into the abyss. Or are we? Does it have to be this way? Can we counteract the effects of aging? Or do we have to accept that we are on a slippery slope? The good news is that our athletic lives don't have to end at our age. Far from it! We can still be strong, look good, and feel great! For example, I recently overheard my very attractive wife (more on her later) describing a young man to her twenty-something daughter. She said, among other things, "But he's not built like Tim." To which my step-daughter rolled her eyes and replied, "Nobody's built like Tim!" I'll admit that I chuckled with pride at my step-daughter's candid, unsolicited observation - she'd *never* say anything like that in front of me! But wait a second! How can that be possible? How can a fifty-something over-the-hill type look and feel better than most guys twenty-five years his junior? Do you have to be a gifted athlete, have super-human genetics, or have been the Big Man on Campus (BMOC)? (If you don't remember that expression, then you're too young for this book!) No, you don't have to fulfill any of the requirements above because the simple fact is that you'll get results if you're dedicated and work hard. The formula for success is good, old-fashioned hard work. No magic potions; no YouTube subscriptions – just you with a proven old-school training program. Quick word-of-caution: you're not about to walk into the gym and pound out the same workout you did thirty years ago. Not in what's left of this lifetime—unless you're thinking of regularly replacing body parts and auditioning for the real-life bionic man. Modification and patience (yes, these terms are unpopular with me too) are the keys to progress. So, how do we make our physical aspirations become, well, more than just aspirations? We'll get there. Promise.

So, who am I and why should you listen to me? I thought you'd never ask! Well, for starters, I've been weight lifting for more than four decades. I was an Olympic-style weightlifter for a few years in my fearless youth. (My parents were ever so thankful that I expressed all my fearlessness on the weightlifting platform and nowhere else!) Before we move on, let me clarify a few things. First of all, I was *never* on an Olympic team. However, I am proud to say that my training partner made the Olympic team in 1980, and I had something to do with it! Secondly, Olympic lifting is a sport featuring two lifts: the snatch and the clean and jerk. (And, if you must know, my best lifts were a 297-pound snatch and a 391-pound clean and jerk. Why the odd numbers? Kilos to pounds, dear reader. Kilos to pounds.) Lastly, Olympic lifting is my first, true love—and yes, my wife has come to grips with that. Back in the seventies (you remember: disco, bell bottoms, and your first color television), my club was a big-time Olympic-style weightlifting club, and a total of four guys made the Olympic team at one time or another. We were a somewhat elitist, competitive club where bodybuilding and bodybuilders were shunned. Strength was king, and little else was on the menu. Our goal was to keep improving our *totals,* which was your best snatch plus your best clean and jerk. Over the years, we'd have fifteen to twenty team members throwing three, four, or even five hundred pounds around every single night. Quite impressive indeed! As my career progressed, five-to-ten ton workouts were the norm—and this did not include the warm-up weights! Standard operating procedure was to have everyone do six to eight sets of their heaviest weight of the night. Out of all this training, I learned one hard-and-fast rule (besides the one about ice really, really coming in handy for sore joints after a workout):

volume is the key to building your body. Volume means to do a lot of sets with a lot of weight. This core principle is as true today as it was back in the day.

"But wait!" you might say. "What does competitive weightlifting have to do with me? All I want to do is get in shape and live to talk about it!" No worries, dear reader. We are going to borrow one of the guiding principles of competitive weightlifting and apply it to our workouts. Also, this book is all about *modification* because if you could do what you did twenty or thirty years ago, you wouldn't need me!

Since my days as a competitive weightlifter, I've tried various workouts over the years, and the pattern I noticed is that when I did a lot of sets of just a few select exercises while staying off most of the machines in the gym, I stayed ahead of the old-age curve. I came to a very straightforward conclusion: simplicity works. I like to keep things simple. Most guys I know like to keep things simple. Simplicity has a profoundness all its own!

Okay, I think we're getting somewhere: simplicity equals sets, reps, and a reasonably heavy weight. This is otherwise known as *volume*. Groovy (you remember that word, right?), but we're forgetting one little thing—the proverbial elephant in the room—we're old. Oh yeah. Now what? Does the bottom falls out? Not by the hairs of your graying chinny-chin-chin it doesn't! The fact that we've lost a little muscle over the years – or, in some cases, a lot - and that most of us have the flexibility of a two by four has been factored into the design of this weight lifting program. We will work around, through, and sometimes, right over these temporary issues. Did you notice that I didn't say *obstacles*? "Patience and modification" doesn't mean we work out like we're made of glass. I'll make you another promise: you will have one of the best - if not *the best* - and most effective workouts in the gym. You will improve faster than you thought possible if you stick with the principles and follow the workouts described in this book. And, you'll be working out the *right* way—a way that will last and last. You only have to promise me and, more importantly, yourself, one thing: you will be patient while undertaking these workout routines. Trying to rush progress or make up for a missed workout is a great way to get injured. I should know because my youthful impatience had devastating, life-long consequences.

Personal Story

As you may have guessed, I was an aspiring Olympic-style weight lifter. My training partner had made the Team, and I was in a great club surrounded by inspiring figures. I was a reasonably good athlete so I thought a spot on the Olympic team seemed possible. In my mid-twenties, I was on my way to getting pretty strong. I had already squatted 500 pounds for five reps and making short work of it, I might add. So, I was moving along nicely. Enter stupidity. One week, I had missed my heavy squat day, which always fell on a Saturday, a non-work day, a day in which I was always well-rested. So to catch up, I thought I'd just squat during the week (after a long work day, a day in which I was far from well-rested). My twenty-five-year-old rationale was that I wasn't going *that* heavy anyway. My workout actually seemed to go pretty well because I achieved my objective, which was 435 pounds for three sets of five reps easily that night. The next morning, I could barely move my left leg because I had partially torn my patella tendon. One workout. One mistake. And my weightlifting career was over—just that fast. Oh sure, I tried to make a comeback. I even squatted 440 pounds for reps at one point. But my abilities were never quite the same. Plus, I was young. We're old. We're not going to make a similar mistake now. We need to have patience in order for our bodies adjust to the new routines. We can always lift that heavier weight tomorrow or next week.

My final word and then we get to the good stuff: I've done everything - and I do mean *everything*! - that I recommend in this book. Over years and years, these routines have been time-tested, juggled, massaged, torn apart, and put back together. I've made every mistake in the book—and some that aren't in the book. The exercises that don't produce results have been thrown out, and the good stuff has been thrown in. I know one thing about these routines: done right, they work! Simple.

Chapter II
Muscle Groups and the Athletic Body

A skinny guy is doing curls; another guy is wrestling with the cables; and another one is grunting on the leg extension machine. Ah, the sights and sounds of a modern gym! Most of the things you see people do in a gym are a waste of time, Yes, performing isolation exercises, working small muscles, and pushing and pulling on the latest machine will *never* produce the results gym-goers so doggedly seek. Never. You simply can't develop your overall physique by working small muscles individually or by doing highly specialized exercises. Ain't gonna happen. Most gym-goers work relatively small muscles with correspondingly light weight or perform exercises that attack a narrow area of the physique, and then they wonder why their body hasn't changed much – if at all. So, unless you have a Mr. Olympia contest in a couple weeks, throw those exercises out and forget they ever existed! Instead, we'll focus on building your base and expanding from there. Working your muscles in groups through "compound exercises" (e.g. your arms, back, and shoulders) will develop your muscles as a unit. In other words, we'll get your muscles all working together - kind of like a team. This will help you achieve the symmetry you desire. I can hear it now: "Yeah but Arnold did curls!" Indeed, he did. He was also a world class athlete in swimming and weightlifting before he ever started body building, so he had a base from which to develop his celebrated physique. The fact is that most people waste their time in the gym. Period. You won't be one of them. Promise.

Pick up your average bodybuilding book or magazine, and what do you see? Hundreds of exercises, "routines of the stars," and Mr. America's latest chest workout. Is it any wonder why people wind up wasting their time in the gym? Cables, flyes, rows, smith machines, decline bench presses, pullovers, planks, lunges, dumbbells this and dumbbells that … OMG … Whiskey-Tango-Foxtrot! Remember, let's keep it simple people! We like simple. The best advice I can give you is to drop the magazines and turn off that bodybuilding website. Let other people waste their time.

Personal Story
Core principle/story time: When I first started Olympic weightlifting, my mentors imparted their core philosophy on me: technique first, strength second, bodyweight third. Okay, to a novice, that principle sounded intriguing. But what exactly did it mean? Basically it meant that, for the first few months of training, I would learn ***how*** to do an exercise, which meant using a broomstick while learning the tough stuff: pulls, cleans, etc. This proposition was a difficult one for an eighteen-year-old former all-state football player with a Type A personality to accept. But I wasn't about to argue with guys who could clean and jerk two of me. After a while, I graduated from the broomstick to the bar, then to weights, and I was on my way! The message was clear: learn the right techniques, and you will be able to lift more weight while avoiding injuries. Eventually, I really understood their method and their madness - and you will too. So let's break it down.

Technique
Proper technique is *absolutely critical* for you to be successful in weight training. Critical. Most of the technique I see from those attempting to use barbells is truly cringe-worthy. They're accidents waiting to happen. That statement may sound a bit elitist but one of my goals is to help you become technically proficient. I want you to be so good at executing proper technique that you'll be able to notice the slightest flaw in your own movements, and you'll be able to correct it on the spot. You'll become, as we used to say,

a "technician." "Yeah, Tim, that's all very well," you may say. "But I just want to get in shape. I'm not a lunatic like you!" Fair enough. But you still need to learn proper technique. Riddle me this: when you drive your car, the gas means "go," and the brakes mean "stop," right? This fundamental holds true whether you are driving to the grocery store or on the race track. So, if you screw up the basics, there's a mess to clean up. The same rule applies to weight lifting.

Personal Story
As I mentioned earlier, my training partner made the 1980 Olympic Team. One of the most interesting footnotes to this story was that, during our post-meet, beer-soaked analysis, we figured that he wasn't the strongest lifter in his weight class that day - from a purely raw power point-of-view. We estimated that he was probably the third strongest. So what pushed him over the top? Technique, technique, technique. He was truly a master of his craft. Plus, he had a very good, competitive weightlifting "head." A powerful combination!

Body Strength
If you want to be able to vacuum behind the couch without having to make a subsequent trip to the chiropractor, then you need to make the goal of developing body strength your highest priority. If you want to grow your muscles, you have to tax them. Once you tax your muscles on a regular basis, the transformation begins: last month's "tough workout" becomes this month's warm-up! In the process, you'll be getting stronger, and eventually, leaner. The best way to accomplish this in the shortest amount of time is by working your largest muscle groups through the use of compound exercises. These muscle groups are designed to handle the volume. The trick is to engage your muscles properly through proper exercise selection. Don't worry: I cover proper exercise selection a bit later. This is also the most *efficient* way to work out as you will be regularly killing two or more birds with one stone!

Body Weight
When I referenced *body weight* in the context of Olympic lifting, I was referring to achieving a specific body weight in a particular weight class. Since you are most likely not going to find yourself gracing a weightlifting platform any time soon, you can ignore that specific definition. However, fast forward to our middle-aged bods, we'll see that most of us could stand to drop a couple pounds. The good news is that it doesn't matter whether you have trouble casting a shadow or cast too much of one, you can still develop that symmetrical physique combined with good, old-fashioned body strength by straightening out your diet and incorporating a systematic resistance program.

So what *is* an athletic body? While we all may have different definitions, generally speaking, an athletic body is the one you notice your wife or sweetheart checking out at the pool. Take a look at Michelangelo's (did you know that that was his *first* name?) statue of David. Here is a beautifully proportioned, muscular, not-too-big male statue. If he were a real, live person, you'd think he was a decathlete or, at least, you'd think that he works out. His physique is muscular, balanced, and well-proportioned. "Okay, time out just one minute, Tim," you might be thinking. "There ain't no way I'm going to look anything like Michelangelo's David or anything even close!" First, I would scold you for your poor grammar. Then, I would look straight into your baby blues and ask, "Why not?" "Because I'm over fifty, and I haven't touched a weight since I got married the second time, and I am seventy-five pounds overweight! That's why not!" Time for another reality -check: As I mentioned earlier, I have a very attractive wife. I'm not saying that for brownie points (although I could always use them), she is an honest-to-goodness hottie. She is in her mid-fifties, and she turns heads wherever we go. "I never notice that," she'd say. She is also a breast cancer survivor who made a commitment to herself that she would never let breast cancer discourage her from staying in shape or living a full life. She's now in the best shape of her life. If she can do it, so can you.

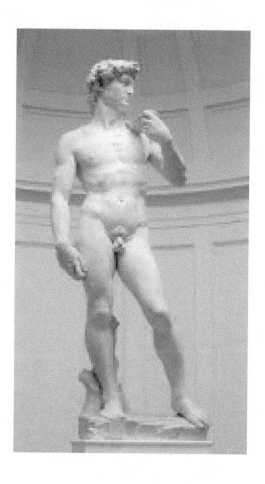

Chapter III
The Preliminaries

The Notebook
We're all a bit egotistical even if we don't want to admit it. We like to look back with pride at some (but Lord knows, not all) of the things we have done over the past few decades. We like to pull out old newspaper clippings in which we were prominently mentioned. We don't mind telling and re-telling that shop-worn story of our famous victory to our spouse or to our significant other. These stories help us keep that I-still-got-it spirit alive, which leads me to my next point. Another vital aspect of your workouts is to keep a diary of your exercises: your sets, reps, and weights. You need to do this a couple of reasons. First, the cliché "it's easier to see where you're going if you know where you've been" applies. Consider it history in the making. If you've ever caught yourself reviewing your Social Security statement and marveling about how you got by on so little income when you were young, you'll know what I mean. When you look back at your notebook after a couple months, you'll find yourself saying things like "gee, two months ago, I could only do *that*?" Then you'll be looking forward to the *next* two months! Second, you're old. You won't remember. Trust me.

Fads. A few words about fads and about that "great workout you saw on the internet!" Okay, I confess: my body is smarter than I am. Don't kid yourself: yours is smarter than you are too! Yes, dear reader, even I, your humble host, have occasionally fallen prey to that "great" chest/shoulder/ab/back workout I saw on YouTube! Hey, I'd like to cheat Father Time too but somehow that never works out. Another case in point: I once fell in love with a so-called beach-body-worthy shoulder routine, which consisted of four exercises in a row, without rest. I admit that I was a bit envious of the shoulders on the guy in the video and pictured myself squeezing sideways through the doorway after doing this workout for a while. "Yes," I thought, "that could be me!" The first time I tried this workout, I was hooked! My shoulders got a great pump, and I could barely get my shirt off to show my wife! Wow! I was hot stuff—even the doorways started to look a bit narrower! Do you know how long that lasted? Exactly two workouts. Yes, *two*—before my shoulder joints started biting back and my elbow began crying. Oh yes, I tried to tough it out: "C'mon, Tim," I said. "You have forty years of experience, and you've been through much worse—like the time 405 pounds fell on your back!" (Another story for another time). But it was all to no avail. My body was unconvinced and, once again, it proved to be much smarter than I am! Needless to say, I bathed myself in ice for a few days, put my tail between my legs, ditched that great beach-body-worthy workout, and got back on track.

Dress Code
When choosing gym wear, you should never "dress to impress." Be mindful of the fact that your clothes are simply another tool to help boost your performance, and you should use them that way. You'll go a long way if you develop the mindset that *everything* you do in the gym will either move you forward or push you backwards. Stick with loose-fitting T-shirts, shorts, and when the occasion calls for it, sweats because you need to stay warm throughout your workout.

Equipment
Remember our plan to keep things simple? We're going to keep things *real* simple here. For the weight lifting routines in this book, you'll need a barbell, a couple of dumbbells, another accoutrement or two, and that's it. You'll be working large muscle groups so you can pass on the preacher curl bench, the leg extension machine, the cables, the smith machine, and the multitude of other stuff you'll find cluttering the

gym. If you work out at home like I do, then you'll need a few other things: a leg press of the vertical or the forty-five-degree-angle variety, a bench that will also incline, a lat machine, and a place to do pull-ups. That should cover it. I've had my "newest" stuff for over twenty years. I bought my bench forty years ago, and it still works just fine. Around that time, I sawed a couple pieces off an old barbell to make the dumbbells that I still use! Invest in good equipment, and you only have to buy it once!

A word about barbells: Barbells will be the most important pieces of equipment in your gym. No other piece of equipment will help you develop both your body and your *balance* as well as the good old-fashioned barbell! Yes, this olden-day invention has yet to be eclipsed as *the* training tool. Whether standing, sitting, or lying down, you must engage your ancillary muscles, which are the muscles that aren't being directly worked, in order for you to maintain your balance while you complete your movements. When you use barbells, you get a complete workout that machines simply cannot match.

How To Use That Belt. Belts are another important piece of equipment to have on hand. Like any other tool, there's a right way and a wrong way to use this one too. And, not surprisingly, most people misuse weight belts as well. Using a weight lifting belt actually takes a bit of coordination. "Really, Tim?" you say. "Now I know you're losing it!" Stick with me here, and I'll explain. Put the belt on so that it's snug around your waist. So far, nothing new. Now, here's where the "coordination" part comes in: push your stomach *out* strongly against the belt while simultaneously arching your back. This creates a solid foundation from which to lift, and it helps keep that back tight! It's tricky, but once you get the hang of it, your technique, and then your weights will improve.

Sets, Reps, and Rest

Gosh, I've heard it all: thirty-second rest! Only do sixty seconds of rest between sets, max! Circuit this and circuit that! Train to failure! Go heavy or go home! Yeah baby! Watch me break a bat over my head! Okay, I made up that last one, but frequently, the gym-goer's mindset is to appear macho. We need to slow down a bit. I promise you that you *will* be challenging your body. Over and over and over again. At the same time, you will be doing so in a way that will leave you looking forward to your next workout; you won't be making up excuses as to why you "just can't find the time." So what *is* the right number of sets and reps, and what is the appropriate rest period? Well, the answer is this: it depends. It depends on where you are in your training, what exercise you're doing, how heavy you're going, and, sometimes, how much time you have to work out. Generally speaking, you'll start out doing three sets of each exercise to start out. The reps and rest periods are going to vary. If you continue on to my advanced routines, you'll move to eight sets for most of the exercises (remember that *volume* concept?). And, again, the reps are going to vary. Also, count on a two-to-four-minute rest period between sets. Final Note: be *precise* with your rest periods. If your workout calls for a two-minute rest period, make it *exactly* two minutes. I wear a watch with a second hand when I work out in a gym so I can keep track of time.

Stretch

Every now and then, we all long for the quick fix, the magic pill that will "make it all better" and solve whatever problem we're facing. When I first started lifting, I remember thinking that if I worked out really, really hard for *one day*, I'd come upstairs from my basement gym looking like a world champion bodybuilder. Youth. Well, I think it's safe to say that the Captain America-type transformations only happen in the movies. Like most things in life, progress is a cumulative thing. The same goes for the most important pre-workout activity you can do: stretching. I'll confess that I was never a big fan of stretching; I've always longed for a flexibility pill myself. The anticipated discomfort with that first stretch always made me look for one or two other things to do before I got started. Once you do get started, though, things start to happen: the body starts feeling suppler, the juices start flowing, and, darn it, you do feel just a bit more athletic! Stretching makes a huge difference in your *mental* workout game too.

So how do we get started? It's always better and easier to stretch warm muscles rather than relatively cold ones. A great way to get going is to first do a few minutes on a stationary bike or calisthenics like jumping jacks, jogging in place, or jumping rope. Anything will work as long as you get the heart pumping warm blood to your cold muscles. Also, make sure that you stretch your *entire* body before each workout. As you'll see in the more advanced sessions, the workouts are split between upper-body days and lower-body days. When you get to that point, you'll be tempted to stretch just the body parts that you'll be working. However, keep in mind that, in addition to preparing you for your workout, stretching is also therapeutic, and it prepares the unit that is resting for the next day's workout. I've outlined some good stretches below.

A. The Arm Swing - Rotate each arm one at a time in wide circles. Do these rotations for a specified time, i.e. for fifteen to twenty seconds at a time; that way you can't cheat. Continue back and forth for one full minute.

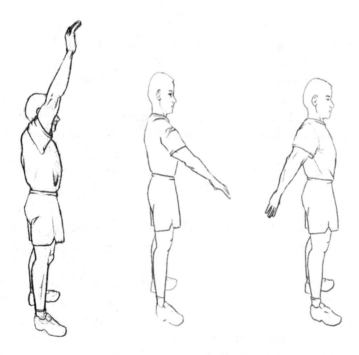

B. The First Shoulder Stretch - Fold one arm across your chest, grab your elbow, and pull gently. Hold that position for five to ten seconds. Repeat the stretch with the other arm. Continue for about a minute.

C. The Second Shoulder Stretch - Point your elbow to the ceiling as vertical as you can, and touch the back of your neck. Allow a second or two for your head to clear. Grab your elbow and pull gently. Remember, this stretch isn't intended as a contest to see how far you can go. The best stretching is controlled stretching. Stretching enables you to maximize your range of motion and help you remain injury-free. Don't skimp, but go slowly.

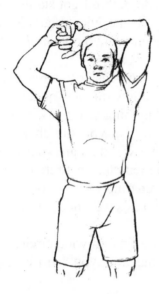

More Great Advice: When stretching, start with your weak side first. If you're righty, start with your left side; if you're lefty, start with your right side. I remember the first time I read this one, and quite frankly, I was a bit skeptical. To my black-and-white way of thinking, it just made no sense that starting with my weaker side would make a dime's worth of difference. So, of course, I put it off. But, at the time, my left hamstring was very tight, and I could never get it real loose no matter what I did or how hard I tried. Nothing worked. So I finally gave it a shot. Within one session—*one session*—I noticed a difference! Now, finally, both legs are in sync, and I no longer favor my left side when I work out.

D. The Pec Stretch - Sounds like this would go good with Punkin' Chunkin'. Find a convenient doorway, or go to the corner of a room. Place your hands on either side of the doorframe, or place one hand on each wall, and lean in *slowly*. Always, always, always do this one slowly. You risk straining your shoulder if you attack this stretch too aggressively—no need to be Rambo here. When you start to feel a good pull, pause for a few seconds. Repeat this exercise a few times until your chest feels stretched out.

E. Overall Leg Stretch - This next exercise is great for your body as a whole; think of it as kind of a group stretch. This stretch will loosen your back, your sides, and, of course, your legs. Sit on a carpeted floor with your feet as far apart as possible and lean forward for a few seconds. Turn towards your weaker leg, hold onto your ankle or foot and gently pull. Eventually, your objective will be to touch your nose to your knee while keeping your leg straight. Repeat this stretch on your strong side. Once you've gone back and forth three times, lean straight forward as far as you can. Hold this position for ten to twenty seconds. Release slowly. Repeat the whole process three times. This stretch feels horrible at first, but your body will feel a healthy "rush" when you're finished! Finally, I recommend stretching in stockinged feet.

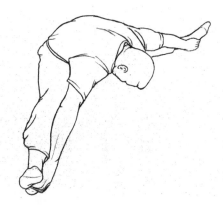

F. Quad Stretch - Let's not forget the quads. Yes, you have to stretch those too! Sit on your lower legs with your hips touching the floor—or at least, try to touch your hips to the floor. Now comes the good part: sit bolt upright and don't slouch. Instead, arch your back—you'll be doing a lot of back-arching when you start the weight lifting exercises so you might as well get used to it. Lean back and hold this position for fifteen to thirty seconds.

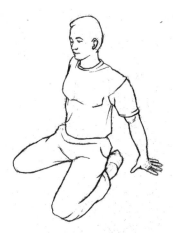

As with the rest of this program, give yourself time to work into each position. We older folks tend to tighten up more quickly than we did once upon a time, so patience is the order of the day!

Chapter IV
The Right Moves

One very important thing to keep in mind while you're working out is that weight training and weight lifting is a lot like dancing: no one notices you unless you're doing the moves really well or really badly. Because you are going to learn how to do all your exercises the right way and you are going to stay focused on your notebook, technique, sets and reps, you won't feel the least bit self-conscious in the gym. If anything, after a while, people will be learning from *you*!

Before you start the exercises I've outlined below, I want to say a word about breathing, which is always a good idea but here's how to apply it as a technique when working out: inhale quickly on the easy part of the lift, i.e. when lowering the weight, and exhale strongly during the hard part of the exercise, i.e. when pushing up the weight. Do not hold your breath! Your muscles need a fresh supply of oxygen to work at an optimum level.

A. Bench Press - We're going to start with an old classic. You've seen just about everyone do this one, and just about everyone does it wrong! Yes, this simple lie-down-flat-and-push-up exercise is butchered by most everyone. The first mistake is the instruction to lie down flat. Then the average bench presser's feet are going in every direction. Lying down flat does not produce much of a base. Would you prefer to build your home on a bed of sand or on a bed of granite? "Granite. Duh, Tim," I can hear you say. Right. So here's how you're going to build a strong base from which to perform this exercise. First, lie on the bench and get your eyes dead even with the bar. For now, start with a grip a bit wider than your shoulders. Now, here's the good part—the part that is going to make your base rock solid—pull your face close to the bar and, at the same time, arch your back as hard as you can. Remember, the more you stretch, the better you'll be able to hold this position. By the way, you're going to want to stretch between sets too, to keep your back nice and limber. Once you have a strong arch, come back down to the bench. Now, walk your feet towards you so that your feet are just past your knees. Finally, push your feet *very hard* into the floor. The only body parts that should be touching the bench are your upper back and your rear end—and that's all. Forget about that "lying flat" stuff. You want to feel as though you are looking up at the bar, almost as if you were on a decline. You're now ready to go. Once you get the hang of it, you'll notice the bar start jumping off your chest!

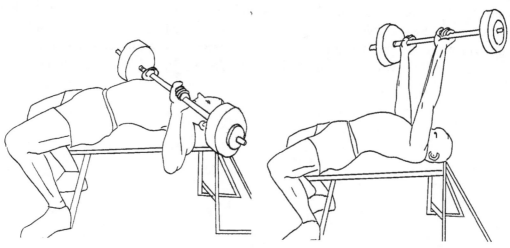

Now for the push-up part of the lift. This technique is a bit unconventional and somewhat counterintuitive. The push-up part of the lift is actually a shallow arc that starts just above the nipple-line and finishes almost in line with your nose. The reason for this arc is that this trajectory keeps the weight over your center of gravity and keeps your largest and strongest muscles engaged throughout the entire movement. Otherwise, if you push it straight up, you will be pushing the bar *away* from your center of gravity, and you will overstress your shoulders. Even if you are an experienced lifter, break your weights down and take the time to re-learn this lift. Your physique and body strength will improve dramatically once you've mastered it.

B. Dips - For this exercise, you get a break from the technique lecture. This one is rather straightforward, and here's what you do: begin the exercise with your arms fully extended. Slowly bend your elbows with your upper body leaning slightly forward. In the full-stretch position, your upper arms should be parallel to the floor. Push hard, keeping your head up, and come back to a vertical position. Make sure you lock your arms out fully each time. As in all of these exercises, the reps should be done in a controlled fashion. Slow down if your hips begin to swing.

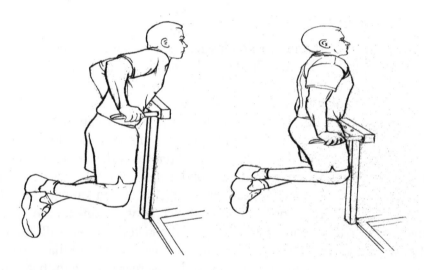

C. Dumbell Bench Press - The way you set up your body in this exercise is very similar to that of the bench press, only you are using a set of dumbbells. You know: arch the back, move the feet, and push through the floor. You will be on a flat bench and the range of motion is exactly the same as it is with the bench press, i.e., a shallow arc from just above the nipples to just below the nose. In order to get the most out of this exercise, keep your hands a good twelve to eighteen inches apart when your arms are fully extended. This hand positioning will put extra pressure on your pectoral muscles, not allowing them to rest. If you have difficulty holding that position with all your reps, reduce the weight so that you can complete all the reps properly. Technique first!

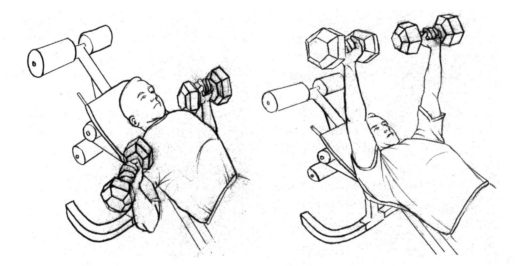

D. Military Press - Take a walk down memory lane for a minute and look at the weightlifters from the forties, fifties, and sixties - you can even find some grainy videos on YouTube. Back then, the military press was a competitive lift, and the competitors would regularly press hundreds and hundreds of pounds. You'll see that these guys had really impressive arms and shoulders! And, yes, their technique was exceptional. (Eventually, in the seventies, the lift was dropped from competition because everyone cheated so badly—using knee kicks and leaning back excessively—none of which you will do!) "Yeah," you say, "that's great for them but I'm not about to press hundreds of pounds!" Relax, grasshopper, you won't have to lift hundreds in order to develop well-rounded and envied-by-others deltoids. This exercise is one of *the* premier exercises as it engages your arms, shoulders, and back in a big way! It's a real strength builder and body toner that no one does these days—maybe because "it's so forty years ago!" Not anymore; we're bringing it back in style. Done properly, you will notice a ***huge*** difference in your appearance in a relatively short period of time because barbells have a way of accomplishing that. However, you have to be careful not to become over-zealous with this one. Don't attempt this exercise until you have a good six-months of weight training under your belt (we used to call that "backlog") as you need a stable base from which to press. You are going to perform this exercise seated at first because the seated version allows you to regroup between reps. Standing forces you to do one press right after the other, which can lead to improper technique - you knew I was going to say that - which can lead to injury.

Okay, here we go! Get a solid chair or a bench and place it *inside* the power rack, which will help prevent an accident if you lose your balance. Don't poo-poo this as lifting accidents happen even to the most experienced lifters. Yes, I'm speaking from experience…

Personal Story
In the summer of 1980, my training partner was fresh off his victory at the Olympic Trials. We were all feeling really good, and I got the bright idea of trying his shoes (he had really cool Russian weightlifting shoes). I figured that if they were good enough for him, they were certainly good enough for me. Unfortunately, I didn't know that the soles were pretty worn, i.e. slippery from months and months of hard training. So, even though they were one size too small, I squeezed into them anyway. I was doing overheads (split jerks) from the power rack. Key Note: the heavier you go, the wider you have to split your feet. I must say that I was pretty good at this lift as I had only missed two overheads in competition in my *entire* career!. The lifts were going along smoothly: 315, 365, 385 and then to 405 pounds, which would tie my personal best. I tightened up, took the bar off the rack, dipped, split quickly and near disaster struck! As

my feet landed, the slippery sole took my rear foot out from under me! I fell over sideways, the weight crashed to the platform, bounced, and landed on my back as I lie face down! An accident that couldn't have looked worse. The place went silent. My teammates froze and turned white. Was I hurt, crippled, both? Before they had a chance to move, I got up, dusted myself off, and shrugged. "Slipped." Being the block-head that I was, I stripped the bar to 225, power-cleaned it, put it back on the rack, loaded it to that 405, changed shoes, and, to the chagrin of my head-shaking teammates, jerked the 405 pounds! Even I have to roll my eyes at that one! The point is that I was a very experienced lifter and *still* had a nasty accident. Don't think it can't happen to you and be sure to take all the necessary precautions to be safe in the gym.

Back to the military press: now that your chair or bench is inside the power rack, adjust the rack so that the bar is about shoulder height when you're seated. Sit very close to the bar with your Adams-apple up against it. Move your feet under your body and arch that back. Put your palms up, elbows slightly forward of the bar, and chin down, and then press straight up forcing your elbows out at the hardest part of the press, which is called the *sticking point*. When in the final position, the weight should be directly over your ears—not too far forward and not too far backward. You'll want to keep the weight light for a while until this movement becomes second nature. Stretch your back between sets here too. A good variation on this exercise is the standing military press, which should only be done after you have mastered the seated press. The move is basically the same except that you'll want to tense your thighs and glutes as hard as you possibly can to lock that lower body in a powerful position from which to press. You'll be tempted to lean back as the weight gets heavier, which is fine as long as you don't over-stress your muscles.

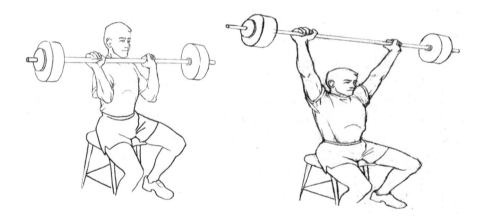

E. Alternate Press - This exercise is a great complement to the military press. You'll do this one on an alternate day because, well, we don't want your shoulders to think we forgot about them. You'll perform this one seated as well in order to isolate your upper body and to reduce the cheating factor. The technique here is very similar to that of the military press: keep your back arched, your head up, and your feet under your body as you push into the floor. Lift the dumbbells to your shoulders and alternately press each one. Remember to start with you weaker arm as it helps you focus better.

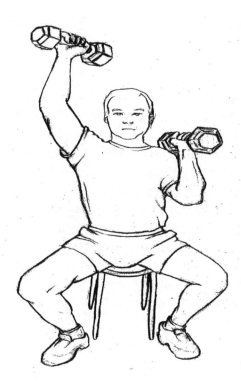

F. Upright Rows - This exercise is another way to develop your shoulders, trapezius muscles, and arms simultaneously—this time from a slightly different angle. Grab that barbell with your palms facing your body, spreading your hands eight to twelve inches apart. Stand up, curl your wrists inward, and bend slightly forward at the waist. Pull the weight up to neck-level, keeping your elbows high during the entire movement. Lower the weight *slowly*. This last point is very important for two reasons. First, slowing the move down will keep your muscles working during this important part of the lift, and second, it will also keep you from lowering the weight too fast or crashing in the finished position, which can result in a lower back injury.

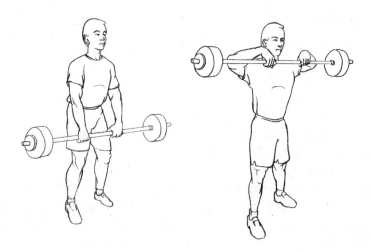

I realize that all this minute detail about how to perform each exercise may seem a bit nutty. We used to have seven or eight key things to remember—shoulders down, elbows out, wrists curled in, back tight, etcetera—before we even lifted the bar! So, focusing on the details of each movement will enable you to perform the move correctly and enable your workouts to be far more effective in the long run. It'll also help keep the injury-bug away. Proper technique is *the* most important component of a successful training program!

G. Pull Downs - This exercise is actually a precursor to your pull-up routine. This exercise is great because it works your arms, back, and shoulders and helps build a well-rounded, athletic physique. Now, you can finally relegate the curl bar to the dust bin (we used to derisively call curls "baby work"). You won't need any isolation exercises, such as curls or triceps extensions, once you implement this entire training program. Keep in mind that once you're strong enough to perform pull-ups regularly, you can put this exercise in the back of the file too; you won't need it anymore. If you're a relative novice, consider this exercise as a stepping stone. And, yes, there's a right way and a wrong way to do this one too. The main key is to keep a tight frame (i.e. keep your back arched, sit as upright as possible, and only pull the weight down *in front* of your neck, not behind your neck). Years ago, most of us were taught to pull the bar behind the neck because it supposedly isolated the back muscles better. Whether or not this claim is true is debatable. What they didn't tell us (and probably didn't know) is that pull-downs behind the neck put an extra, unnecessary strain on the shoulder joints, which is the last thing we need at our age. Use a wider-than-your-shoulders grip and go to town.

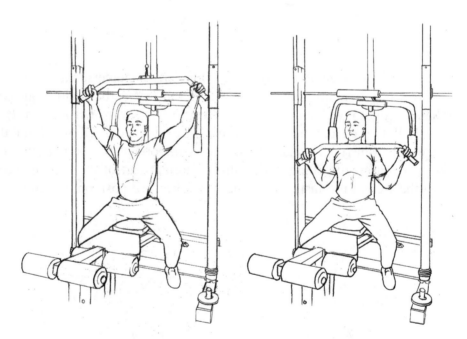

E. Pull-ups - This exercise is one of my personal favorites! This simple (remember, we like simple) yet tough exercise is a fantastic strength builder and muscle builder. With its endless iterations, it renders most of the other back exercises obsolete, and yet so few focus on it because it's difficult, and it takes time to work into a routine. Because you can perform this one in a number of different ways, it will become one of your foundational exercises. If you have experience in weight lifting, you'll be able to dive right into it. If you're a beginner, then you'll need to develop some basic strength first. Depending on where you are in your workout plan, you can do the exercise with your palms facing forward, with your palms facing in towards your ears, which is my favorite, or with your palms facing your body. As you begin to work pull-ups into your routine, start doing them with your palms facing away from you. You can work the other variations in as your training progresses. The biggest thing you have to worry about while doing this exercise is cheating; make sure you are extending your arms fully between reps and do not kick your feet.

F. Leg press - Practically every fifty-plus-year-old man is derided (behind his back, of course) for his "chicken legs." Arguing with that statement is kind of difficult since skinny legs poking through a pair of shorts or from a bathing suit is a fairly common sight for the fifty-and-over crowd, and those skinny legs *do* have a certain ostrich-like look to them. Legs typically are the most neglected part of the anatomy. The reason for this is simple: leg work is tough, grueling, and un-sexy. You'll never find a crowd around the squat rack or the leg-press machine.

Personal Story

I was in my early forties when I began dating my wife-to-be. We had come back to her place after shopping (Yes, I was quickly being indoctrinated), and she mentioned something about me having a "flat ass" (!), which wasn't the case, by the way. Well, you all know that the scourge of getting older is losing the round glutes, and I went into full-on, *panic* mode! I cancelled the rest of our day, went home, and leg pressed like a maniac! No way was I losing my round ass! Later, my back-tracking sweetheart insisted that all was round with my hind-quarters, but she delighted in the fact that she found a way to send her weight-lifter boyfriend into a stampede of frenzied vanity!

Getting back to the leg press....: flexibility is the *key* to the leg press. So, prior to your leg workout, make sure that you stretch for an extended period of time. There are two important things to remember when completing this movement. First, keep your hips in contact with the leg press sled. Do not allow them to ride up and round your lower back as this can cause lower-back strain. Second, keep your toes and, more importantly, your knees pointed out. This position allows you to engage the hips more fully and keeps the pressure off the knees. Resist the temptation to bow your knees inward as it can really damage your knees.

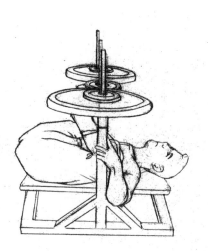 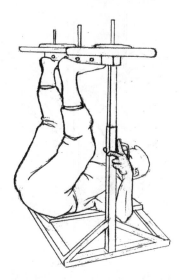

G. Calf Work - The section below the knee rarely, if ever, gets a good workout. Yes, we're about to change that too! The calf muscles are generally more resistant to change and to development than other body-parts so you have to be persistent. High reps combined with heavy weight is the order of the day. On this one occasion only, I will recommend a machine because it is easy to use, and it isolates these muscles well. Every gym has one of these machines. If you're working out at home, this calf exercise is a bit more complicated to do, but you can still manage. Place the bar on the power rack around knee height, and wrap a pad around the center of the bar. Stand up with it. Step back and sit in a very solid chair while placing the bar on your knees. Now you're ready for heel raises. Go to full contraction, pause for a second, and then come down.

H. Good Mornings - Once upon a time when young men actually had manners, they would greet the female of the species with a courteous bow and a "good morning" (as opposed to a modern-day "What up?"). As you might have guessed, that's where this exercise gets its name—from days long gone—and it involves bending from the waist or "bowing." It strengthens and builds your back's core muscle groups, the erector spinae, which flank both sides of your spine. Over the years, I have seen exactly nobody else do this exercise outside of my wife, whom I taught, and folks in the Olympic weightlifting community. By the way, my wife has perfected this exercise, and it does wonders for her fifty-plus-year-old back! And, while I hate to admit it, she does them better than I do! One day, I was lifting in a gym, and, in the middle of my Good Mornings, a gym's personal trainer asked me what I was doing as he'd never seen or heard of this exercise before. Things that make you go "Hmmm…". Anyway, you'll be doing this one seated as it isolates the back muscles and makes the lift less complicated than doing it standing. The range of entire movement is about eight to twelve inches. "That doesn't seem possible!" you say. "How can a couple of inches do you any good?" Tut, tut. Just try it and see. Here's what you do: with the bar placed *inside* the power rack (remember our discussion about avoiding accidents?), lean underneath the bar and position it across your shoulders. At this point, you'll be in the bottom of the bow. Tighten your shoulder blades together and tighten your lower back *before* you come up to about an eighty degree angle—that is the finishing position, or the top of the bow. You do *not* want to go vertical as you risk doing a "180" and injuring your back. Come back down slowly, touch the rack, and repeat. Do not crash in the bottom. Stretch between sets as well. If you do this exercise consistently, you should be able to lift up to your bodyweight in no time.

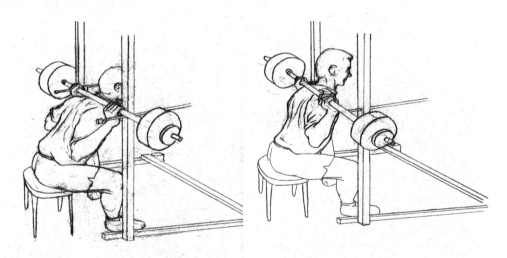

I. Abdominal Exercises - These exercises do not require any "technique talk." Did I just hear a "thank goodness"? We're going to keep this part of our routine pretty simple: we'll do sit-ups and leg lifts. Oh, but there are so many iterations! Lots of different reps, sets, and sequences! You'll feel as though you are doing a different exercise almost every time. When we get to the routines, I'll explain the various ab exercises in more detail, and I promise that you'll never get bored and that your midsection will sting!

Personal Story

My three-year-old granddaughter is my little love—and, sometimes my little training partner. One day, she saw me doing leg lifts and wanted to join the fun. Because I am wrapped around her little finger, I obliged, and taught her how. After a couple of reps, she stopped, sat up and said, "Granddad, don't these hurt your belly?" Only if you do them right, hon.

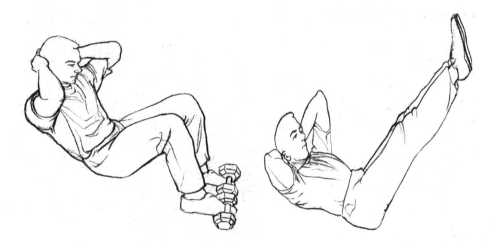

J. The Worst Exercise in the World - My father showed me this exercise over forty years ago, and I'm still mad at him for it. I only started doing the exercise way back when because my older brother was doing it. This exercise is officially called the Wrist Roller but I like my name for it better. What I *do* know is that it is great for the shoulders, forearms, and hands! "Hey," you interject, "I thought you just said you hated it." I do. I really, really do! But it is also very effective. To do this one, you'll need a dowel about two inches thick. Drill a hole through the center of the dowel, and then put a rope about four feet long through the hole and tie a knot. Tie a weight to the other end and, for now, five or ten pounds should be fine. Holding onto the dowel, lift it straight out from your body and "walk" the weight up the rope. When it gets to the top, walk the weight back down. Don't cheat by letting the weight slip to the floor or by lowering your arms. Do this a couple times at the end of your workout. You'll hate me for it, but it's a great last-exercise-of-the-night exercise!

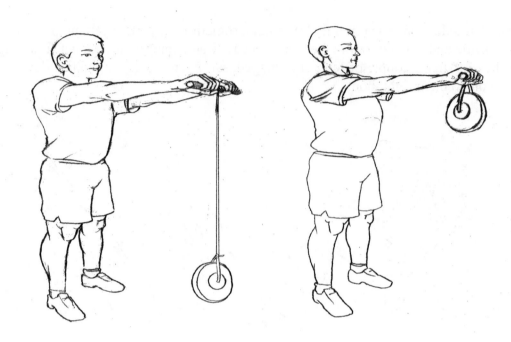

Advanced Moves - Not for the Faint-of-Heart

A. Back Squats - "What do you mean 'advanced'?" you say. "I used to do this exercise in high school!" Yes, well, in all likelihood, you were doing it wrong in high school. Plus, way back when, you could lift with bad technique and your body could shrug it off. Not anymore, old man. My first piece of advice is to look away anytime you see someone doing this lift in the gym. Ninety-nine percent of the time they are doing it incorrectly—most often really, really incorrectly—and you don't want their bad habits to rub off on you. If you ever were to pick a time to be a technique snob, this is it. This exercise involves a number of "moving parts" and it is a difficult lift to master so take lots of time to learn it.

Personal Story

During my first few *years* of Olympic weightlifting, I had been squatting all wrong. I had the weight too high on my shoulders, which caused me to lean too far forward, and I was, essentially, crashing in the bottom of the lift—not a formula for success. Finally, I went too heavy one night and almost severely injured both legs. Only my youth saved me. A good friend, who was also an alternate on the 1980 Olympic team, pulled me aside and finally talked some sense into me, which was not an easy task. I was very fortunate to have been associated with so many talented athletes! Anyway, he broke me down - technique-wise - and we worked on my technique for about six weeks. I was not to go above 340 pounds, which was difficult for me to accept as I had squatted around 475 pounds at the time. This lower weight allowed me to *feel* the movement as we didn't have mirrors in the gym until it became natural. Within another eight weeks, I squatted a career high of 500 pounds for five reps - with this same person spotting me! A very fitting finale'! The moral of the story is that patience pays off. I was an experienced lifter, and learning to squat correctly still took me a lot of time. There is no room for egos here.

For the back squat, you'll want that belt. This piece of equipment will really help you keep your back tight, which is absolutely essential for this lift. Position the bar across the shoulders, *not* on top of the traps. I like to see a line, i.e., the bar, going from the top of one shoulder to the top of the next. Tighten your entire back and lift the bar from the rack. By the way, this is another reason to have a solid backlog of the Good Mornings before you start squatting. Take two steps back while keeping your head up and your knees slightly bent. Shift your hips back, keep your trunk erect, and slowly sink into the bottom position, which occurs when the tops of the thighs are parallel to the floor. "Yeah, right, Tim," you may say. "Good luck getting my body to do that one!" Now you know why I want you to stretch! Reaching the bottom point will take some time, so go as far down as you can while maintaining good form. Trying for that extra inch or two will only cause your back to loosen up, and a round back throws off the entire lift and can result in injury. When you get close to your bottom position, tense your glutes as hard as you can to stop your descent. This facilitates your ascent and helps you keep a tight back. This glute-tightening move will help the lift feel exceptionally smooth. When you reach the top, get ready for the next rep. *Do not bounce.* Bouncing does not look cool, and it only serves to throw you off for your next rep.

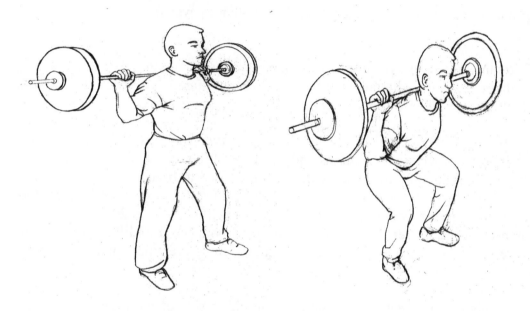

Most people have real problems getting the technique for the back-squat right. Here are a few technical points for you to remember:

1. Shifting the hips is *essential* to getting this technique down properly because it places the hips in line to handle the burden of the weight.
2. The bar must be placed on your *shoulders,* in a line going across your back, in order for you to maintain a good position. If you place the bar too high, e.g. on the traps, you will lean forward, which can cause both knee and lower back problems. If the bar is placed too low, e.g. like in a power lifter's stance, you lose the benefit of developing your thighs, which, of course, is the whole point of this exercise.
3. The knees should *never* go beyond or over the toes in the bottom position. If they do, it's a good indication that you are leaning too far forward. When you hit the bottom, the front of your knee should be even with the tip of your toes.
4. The bar should remain in line with your ankles during the **entire** move. This provides you with the optimum mechanical advantage.
5. Never completely straighten your legs during this lift. You *always* want your muscles to support the weight—not your joints!

6. When you reach the *sticking point* on the way up, which is usually about half way up, force your knees out and your hips in. This trick will really help when you start to go heavy!

High-Tech Piece of Advice: use your phone to record each set. This is a great training tool and will help you immensely. Your persistence will pay off, and you will learn it correctly!

Personal Story
When my training partner started Olympic lifting, which was several years before I did, his technique was absolutely *horrible*! He was stopping mid-lift, swinging the bar, and jumping back—a coach's nightmare. An Olympian advised the team's coach: "Forget about this guy. He'll never make it." The coach disagreed and worked and worked on this lifter. They worked on strength, technique, mindset—everything. Less than four years later, he was standing on the winner's podium having won the Olympic Trials and tying the American record in the clean and jerk in the process! Persistence pays off.

SPOTTING
I can think of no other aspect of gym-safety more important than spotting. Yet, so many people do this so horribly wrong that I am surprised more people aren't severely injured as a result. *If you learn nothing else from this book, please learn how to spot properly!*

Spotting for the Back Squat: you've all seen the "bear-hug" type spot in which the "spotter' stands *behind* the lifter – usually in his space – with his arms underneath the lifter. Should the lifter fail to complete a rep (we used to call that "getting pinned"), the "spotter" is supposed to bear-hug the lifter and the barbell and help him stand. *This may be the worst idea ever.* Here's why: if the lifter gets pinned, there's usually a good reason such as fatigue or even injury. Let's say that the lifter weights 200 lbs and he's squatting 250 lbs and gets pinned. The "spotter" is now supposed to lift both the tired lifter and the 250 lb weight by himself from a very awkward position. Unlikely. Success here is even more unlikely if the lifter is injured or falls forward.

The Right Way: this requires **two** spotters standing on either side of the lifter. The spotters clasp their fingers together and keep their hands underneath the bar as the lifter moves through each rep. Should the lifter get pinned, the spotters will be able to "catch" the bar and help the lifter back to the squat rack. This technique covers all eventualities: fatigue, injury and even if the lifter falls backwards or forwards.

P.S. Always ask the lifter how many reps he or she will be attempting. This will give you an idea of the lifter's capabilities.

Personal Story
One workout, my training partner was squatting heavy and was going to try to do 455 lbs for 10 reps. He made 9 ½. No big deal. He had two spotters on either side, me and another guy, with our hands ready. When he got pinned, we caught the weight and helped him back to the rack. It was routine and should be.

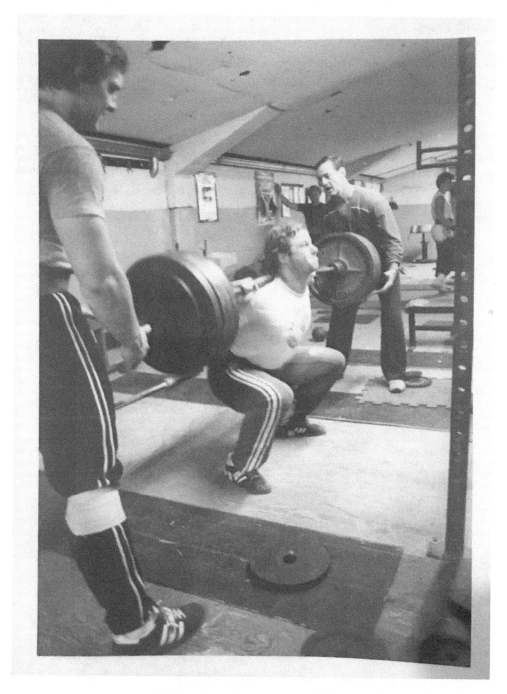

This is how to spot. That's me lifting. The guy on the left was an alternate on the 1980 Olympic Team. The guy on the right was our coach.

Spotting for the Bench Press

For very heavy weights, use the same technique as you would with the back squat. Most of time, the following technique will do: stand at the lifter's head and be sure not to crowd him. Grasp the bar with your palms facing you. Have the lifter tell you when he's ready and on the count of "three", you pull the bar up as the lifter pushes off. You maintain a hold on the bar until the lifter is steady and ready to bench. Let go and take a short step back. Getting out of the way allows the lifter to focus. I find nothing more annoying than to have a well-meaning spotter's crotch in my face as I'm trying to lift. Keep a very close eye on the lifter's progress. If you see him struggling, move in a bit closer but not on top of him. If the lifter gets pinned, you're right there to pull the bar back to the rack. Again, ***always*** ask the lifter how many reps he will be attempting.

B. Front Squats - Once you've mastered the back squat, you'll be able to move into this lift without much of a problem. Developing a base of strength from leg presses and then from back squats is *essential* before you include this exercise as part of your training regimen. This exercise is a great variation that will impact your thighs in a slightly different manner than the back squat. Start by gripping the bar in a position slightly wider than your shoulders and take the weight off the rack with your elbows pointing in front of you. I am an Olympic lifting snob so I prefer this method. However, another method for the tight-in-the-shoulder-joint crowd is to fold your arms like you were "Jeanie" in "I Dream of Genie," place the bar across your shoulders, and put your hands on top of the bar. As long as you keep your elbows extended forward, you'll be able to control the barbell. From there, the lift is the same as the back squat: take two steps back, shift your hips while keeping your upper body erect, and lower yourself into the bottom position. The knees should not go past the toes in the bottom position, and the weight should be over the ankles. Tighten the glutes in the bottom of the lift to control your descent. Keep your elbows high and come back up. If you run into problems, at the sticking point, for example, force your knees outward and pull your hips inward.

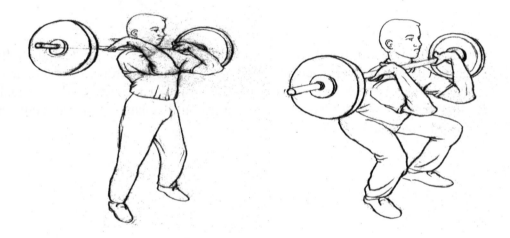

A Word on Wraps. Wraps are another vital tool for us old guys. Actually, wraps transcend age, but the older we get, the more quickly we tend to tighten up, so we need them even more now. Many people harbor the misconception that wraps are used to support, or to take some of the burden off, your joints. Only power lifters use them this way. They tighten their wraps—known as *super wraps*—so tightly that they look like the Michelin Man. We'll only need them to keep our joints *warm*. That's the only reason we use them; no magic involved. Neoprene works best. Keep them snug, but not tight.

C. Inclined Bench Press - This exercise is a bit too advanced for most people. It should be incorporated into your routine only after you have built a solid base. Once again, technique is the key to success. Do you notice a recurring theme here? Set your base *exactly* as you did for the bench press, i.e. arch your back, walk your feet in, and push your feet through the floor. Because of the odd angle on the incline bench, you're going to want to move your feet away from your body a little in order to maintain a better balance. Keep your eyes focused upward as you work; otherwise, you'll have a tendency to push the bar out and away from your center of gravity.

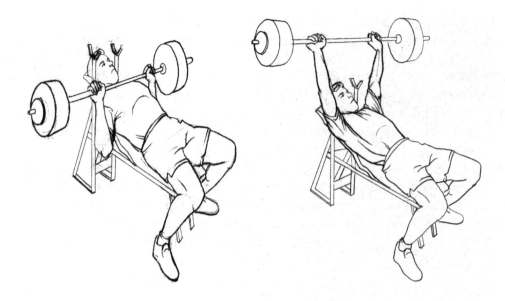

As you apply the exercises described in this chapter, be mindful of our basic tenet: technique first, strength second, and body weight third. Many lifters sacrifice good technique in an effort to boost their weights on a particular exercise. This, however, only succeeds in quickly curtailing progress and, eventually, leads to injury. The one thing that the great athletes have in common is that they have mastered the nuances of their craft. Take the time to learn, and you will soar!

Chapter V
Variations: Time for a Change

Once you've been working out for a while, this section will become the most important part of the book. The main reason people give up working out is that they get bored, or they feel as if they're not getting anywhere: "I've been there; done that. Gee, the game's on. Yawn." Not so anymore. This chapter is where the fun *really* begins, and where I'll show you how to extend these basic routines so they'll last indefinitely. The beauty of this workout philosophy is that only slight variations will make a *huge* difference in your results even though you are doing essentially the same exercises, which is another reason that all those fancy machines in the gym are a waste. A little creativity will propel you to new heights! As you move through your workout cycles, you can begin to make small but significant changes to each exercise. Your workouts can become as creative as you are. I'll give you lots of great ideas—all of which I've tried so I know they work. Your workouts should literally be fun - no, I'm not losing it here! You'll smirk at your own creativity as you know your body is going to be continually challenged in a new and different ways Remember, your body *is* smarter than you are, and it will get very bored, i.e. used to your workout, long before you do. So keep it fresh, and don't hesitate to make a change.

Order

Try shaving the *other* side of your face first, and you'll notice how odd that feels. Well, changing around the order in which you do your exercises will have much the same effect on your muscles. They will feel challenged a bit differently and under constant pressure to adapt. Once your muscles adapt to this change, you can switch your routine back to the way you originally had it, or you can move on to another variation. For example, if you've been doing bench presses followed by dumbbell bench presses, try reversing that order. Once you've done that for six weeks, any change from there will feel like a fresh start for your muscles. Six weeks seems to be the magic number; after six weeks, our bodies figure out what we've been up to, and they adjust accordingly.

Rest Period

This variation is simple and easy to implement. With this one, you don't have to change your exercises, sets, reps, grips, exercise order, or anything else. Your body will feel a new challenge in the form of a shorter, or longer, rest period. So let's say that you've been waiting four minutes between heavy sets (like I do). Reduce that to three minutes and slowly build back up to your normal max weight. Keep in mind that you probably won't be able to handle your four-minute-rest weight right away. You can keep the sets and reps the same. This small change makes the routine a whole new ballgame as far as your muscles are concerned!

Super Sets

This routine is truly not for the faint-of-heart. Super sets transform your routine into both a body-building *and* a cardio workout. A super set involves working one body part and then immediately working a different one. For example, do a set of bench presses and then immediately move on to a set of pull-ups. Wait two to three minutes, and then do another super set. Start with four super sets and work up to six. I guarantee that you *will* huff and puff, but it's awesome! If you really want to go over the top, throw in a set of military presses after the pull-ups. These are called "Tri-Sets. This variation is very effective and should be done only once a week. Otherwise, you'll begin to dread your workouts because super sets are grueling. You can also throw this variation into your routine when you have only a short time to work out. It's a nice feeling sometimes to get through your workout in a half an hour or so and to know that you really accomplished something!

Pre-Exhaustion

Most of us were raised on the following doctrine: "Use heavy weight first, and then move on to a lighter weight." And, that philosophy *is* a very good strengthener and body builder, but it's not the only game in town. When I first tried the pre-exhaustion idea, my parochial mind was throwing a fit: "There's no way this is going to work. It's a dumb idea. Go back to the old way!" Well, as usual, my body was smarter than I was, and the workout was a great success. Now, I use it just about every time I go heavy on the leg press or squats. This variation will help you get a good pump going, which provides a nice cushion around your muscles.

Here's what you do. Let's stick with the leg press example: do a light weight for a high number of reps for a few sets. Then move onto your heavy weight for the day. For example, on a heavy leg press day assuming the target weight is 400 pounds for three sets of five reps, do an Enduro (see Chapter VI) at 200 to 225 pounds. Now your legs should be burning! Jump to 300 pounds for five reps, and then to 400 pounds for the rest of your sets. You can do the same thing on the bench press: do a few sets of dumbbell bench presses with a short rest between sets. Then move on to your regular bench press routine. It really throws your body off! You'll be *amazed* about how differently your body will look and feel after you complete this variation!

One-and-A-Third Reps

So far, all of the routines I've showed you have one thing in common: all the repetitions we've done have been complete movements covering the *entire* range of motion. Most of the time that works well. But you wouldn't want to get bored, would you? Well, this variation is a lot of fun, and it is another great way to challenge your muscles! Again, let's return to our leg press example. Start with your legs fully extended, and then bring the weight down until your legs are fully contracted. Now, instead of driving the weight up fully, drive it only about a third of the way up, bring it back down, and then drive it to full extension. It's another way to strengthen your hips and burn your thighs. Keep the number of sets and reps the same. By the way, you can do this variation on all the exercises described in this book.

Barefootin'

My mother used to tell me that "fingers were made before forks." I'm going to update that saying and apply it to weight lifting by recommending that you remove your shoes and leg press barefoot or, at least, in your stockinged feet. So, my revised saying is "feet were made before shoes." I can hear you balk: "Tim, are you nuts?" While my kids will happily make a case for that, remember that I've done *everything* that I recommend in this book. Everything. So I know it works. While barefooting takes a little getting used to, you'll be rewarded with stronger, more rugged thighs. Leg pressing barefoot stresses your thighs and glutes in a different manner than if you were using shoes. It also engages your ancillary muscles, which aren't normally worked when you're wearing shoes.

Get a Grip

Actually, this section should really be titled, "Change Your Grip," but that's not as catchy. This variation is a very simple one: all you do is change the grip you use while doing bench presses, pull-ups, military presses, leg presses, and so on. Okay, smarty, you do not change the grip per se on the leg press, but you do change the width of your feet. Move your grip either in or out a half-inch to an inch on each side. On the leg press, move your feet either in or out a couple of inches on each side. Do the same number of sets and reps. That small variation changes the entire dynamic of the movement.

Slow Down. Take It Easy.

Okay, I admit that I've employed a little bait-and-switch here. We're going to slow it down, but we're not going to take it easy. Quite the contrary. This variation burns and burns, and it is a fantastic strength and muscle builder. Up until now, all of your reps have been performed steadily—not too fast; not too slow. And, yes, we're about to change that too. Each repetition is going to last four to six seconds, two to three seconds on the way down, and two to three seconds on the way up. Maintain that pace for *all* your repetitions. This variation will be a toughie for you if you're of the fast-twitch-muscle, Type A personality variety. You'll need to really focus to do these right, especially once you get deep into your sets. Do everything else - your sets, reps, exercises, and rest periods - in the same manner as before.

Can you see how effective and simple, yet profound these routines are? The same exercises combined with small but significant variations provide you with an almost infinite variety of new workouts! These new workouts will improve your progress to a level that you didn't think possible. So far, you've learned how to prepare for your workout, how to use the proper technique, and how to build your routines so that they're not, well, routine. I think you've earned a bonus, don't you?

Chapter VI
The Bonus Section

I call all of the exercise in this chapter "achievement workouts" because they make you feel like you've *really* accomplished something when you get through them! Once again, they are not for the faint-of-heart, but you've come this far so I know you can handle it. They are fairly simple (remember, we like simple), yet demanding routines.

Achievement Pull-ups
Do three *maximum* sets with two minutes of rest in between each set. Set a target number of *total* pull-ups you want to complete in order to stay motivated. Do this twice during your normal workout routine, but only incorporate it once a week as your muscles *will* need time to recover!

Ab Work
Go to the mall or to the pool or to any place where a fairly large number of people gather, and count the flat midsections you see on middle-aged men - or any-aged men for that matter! Don't worry about not having enough fingers and toes, and don't worry about bringing a score card—the chances are that you won't need it. "Yeah, well," you say, "the chances that are I won't have a flat midsection anytime soon either, Bub!" Bub? Well, we went from bi-plane to jet during World War II, so I bet we could handle this as well. A flat, tight midsection is well within the realm of possibility; you just have to *decide* to do it. Two changes are required to obtain the flat midsection. First, you have to change your diet, and the best advice I can give you there is to get a book on nutrition as I am by no means an expert on this subject. Second, you have to engage in a workout regimen that challenges your abdominals. I have a couple of good ideas to help you with this goal (you knew I was going to say that), which should be implemented once you have a six-month backlog from the previous workouts.

- Achievement Sit-Ups, Variation #1 - Do three sets of sit-ups as follows: two, two-minute sets of maximum reps, and then one, one-minute set of your maximum reps. Rest for 90 to 120 seconds between sets. This exercise takes a total of five minutes of work. Next, do four sets of leg lifts for ten to twenty reps. Start holding five-pound or ten-pound plates once you've been doing the sit-ups for a while. Also, try holding a light dumbbell between your feet when you're doing your leg lifts. You ask, "What? Do I look like Houdini?" No comment.
- Achievement Leg Lifts, Variation #2 - This variation is basically the same workout as the first variation, except that the *order* of the exercises is reversed. It will feel like a completely new routine because the stress on your abs is a bit different. So, do three sets of leg lifts: one for 2 minutes, one for 2 minutes, and then one for one minute, then do four sets of twenty sit-ups. As you progress, add some weight when doing the sit-ups.
- The Eight-minute Drill, Variation #1 - This exercise is similar to the others, but it attacks your abs in a slightly different fashion. Do one minute of sit-ups, and then immediately do one minute of leg lifts. Hold some light weights while doing the sit-ups. Take a two-minute rest. Repeat this exercise three more times, so you complete eight minutes of work in total. If you're not writhing by the third set, you're doing these exercises incorrectly!
- The Eight-minute Drill, Variation #2 - This variation reverses the eight-minute drill: do leg lifts first, and then sit-ups second. You should now use weights for *both* the leg lifts and the sit-ups.

So now you have four great variations for your abs, and no room for excuses! These workouts are simple, tough, and effective, and I promise that you won't get bored!

Just a Minute
I was doing a little "workout research" a while back and came across this routine. Actually, I've modified this exercise because quite frankly I'm too damned old to do this the right way. As you may know, our Special Forces soldiers have a distinct regimen. One drill that they do to *warm-up* is to do push-ups for two minutes straight! Yes, that's not a misprint. I wasn't going to be able to pull that one off, so I figured I'd modify it a bit and do push-ups for just one minute. It is absolutely killer, a great variation, and a fantastic workout! To be completely honest, I have yet to complete the full minute but I'm getting close! Bring your "A" game to this one!

Enduro
Ah, an oldie but a goodie! My training partner and I customized this one eons ago; it is a Frankenstein-like creation. We started using this one as a light warm-up, but soon, we morphed it into a killer leg routine - and it has stayed that way ever since! It consists of just three relatively light sets of leg presses. Oh, but that darn rest period! Ten seconds between sets. That's it: just ten seconds. So, do twelve reps. Wait ten seconds. Do ten reps. Wait ten seconds. Do eight reps. Collapse. Use lighter weight for this one but don't baby it either. If you're leg pressing 300 pounds for five sets, then use 150 pounds or so for an Enduro.

Special Forces
While I was doing some more workout research, I found this one too. Our Special Forces soldiers do this one too (again, as a warm-up!). You should attempt this one only after you've built a solid base with your pull-ups, sit-ups, and bench presses. You'll need every bit of strength and energy! Here is the routine: one hundred pull-ups, two hundred push-ups, and three hundred sit-ups. Now, don't panic: we split these up into ten sets. "Gee, that really helps, Tim," you might say dripping with sarcasm. Well, it does get a little better - but not much: you can rest two minutes between sets. So, do ten pull-ups, twenty push-ups, and thirty sit-ups in rapid succession. Then rest two minutes and repeat. Nail that ten times, and you're done! Easy. The material I read concerning this workout didn't specify a rest period, so I suspect that the Special Forces personnel are required to do this exercise *without* rest. Yikes! Thank God they're on *our* side! By the way, I once tried this workout during my week off, which was a really dumb idea (so don't do it). Instead, use this routine when you feel need a change during one of your regular workout weeks.

The Two-minute Drill
I heard or read somewhere that our Marines do this workout. If that's true, it's really cool; if not, we can always pretend that they do it. This one's a toughie, but if you've come through the advanced program and are looking for a good variation, you can settle in right here. This workout encompasses a lot of pull-ups, i.e., forty, in a small amount of time: two minutes. Yes, forty pull-ups in two minutes—you read that right. Before you skip this one, remember that you can do more than you think you can. I am not going to share any stories with you although a couple come to mind, but I *am* speaking from experience. One tip: don't try to do two sets of twenty in two minutes because that probably won't work. I recommend that you split this up into two sets: do your maximum amount of pull-ups, wait about sixty seconds, and then do the rest. When you get really good, try this one a couple of times in one night. For now, once should be enough!

Chapter VII
Basic Training

You've come this far, and I hope you've learned a thing or two besides the fact that it's a miracle that I've lived so long. You've reached the "workout" part of the book, a.k.a. where the rubber meets the road, the acid test, or the [*please feel free to insert your own motivational action phrase here*]. Your workouts are designed to be both efficient and effective. "Wow. Great slogan, Tim," you say, "but what on earth are you talking about?" Here's what I mean: your workouts will be *efficient* because you will work a lot of muscle *groups* with just a few exercises; your workouts will be *effective* because we are going to build *volume* into your routine. You will make the most progress in the shortest amount of time by consistently working large muscle groups through the use of compound exercises, and, by the way, you'll also be spending the least amount of time in the gym necessary to build a first-class physique! Your workouts are going to be built around a few core exercises, which work over eighty-five percent of the muscles in your body! Think about that: a few exercises cover eighty-five percent of your muscles. The goals of strengthening and sculpting are compacted in one nice, neat little package! Simple plus well-conceived workouts equals effective training.

If you're comfortable staying at the beginner stage, for example, then by all means, stay there. You can still make great progress at that level as long as you vary the exercises in some form or fashion. I'll discuss these variations at length a bit later.

Warm-ups
Before you begin any of these workouts, remember to do both the stretching exercises and the warm-ups we discussed as

The Beginner Workout
If you haven't touched a weight in a long time because of the kids' softball, baseball, band, chorus, soccer, swim meets , or basketball games or if you've just been dabbling in the gym, then you should start with this beginner workout. You're going want to work into this routine gradually in order to avoid soreness and deter that urge to say, "Gee, I just can't make it to the gym for the next part of my life."

Personal Story
I started my twenty-something-year-old son on this routine. Although he was not a regular in the gym, I figured that because of his age, he could dive right into the three-day per week, multiple-set routine. Oops. About two weeks after he started, I texted him (yes, I've made it to the twenty-first century!) to see how he was doing. Well, he hadn't made it to the gym in a few days because of "killer soreness." The moral of the story is that it's best to start off slowly before you hit the gas.

This routine is deliberately designed to feel as if you're proceeding at a "snail's pace". This pace is a good and appropriate speed to start your weight training because it'll keep you looking forward to your next workout. This routine is designed to last for three months, but it will be split up into two six-week parts.

The First Six Weeks

Do the following routine two days per week to start and do it this way for six weeks. You need a minimum of two days of rest between workouts. So a Monday/Thursday or a Tuesday/Friday routine will be just fine.

- Pull Downs (palms facing forward): three sets of ten reps.
- Bench Press: three sets of five reps.
- Alternate Dumbell Press: three sets of ten.
- Leg Press: three sets of ten reps.
- Sit-ups: three sets of twenty reps. (Do not use any weight.)

Yes, that's it. Don't push for an extra set, additional reps, or another exercise. Also, do them in the order described above and wait three minutes between sets. Keep in mind that all three sets *must* be done with your final weight. Warm ups *do not count!* So, if 200 pounds is your final weight on the leg press, for instance, your warm-ups with 100 pounds and 150 pounds do not count towards the three sets. In this example, you would need to do three sets of ten with 200 pounds. You're starting to build volume into your workouts!

The Second Six Weeks

Add a day to your workout routine and go Monday, Wednesday, and Friday.

Wednesday's Workout: *Always Very Light*

- Chest Flyes: 3 x 10
- Pull Downs: 3 x 8
- Shoulder Flyes: 3 x 10
- No Legs – give them a break. They'll need it.

While I realize that this doesn't seem like much, it'll keep your body stimulated and facilitate conditioning.

Monday and Friday: keep the exercises, sets, rest periods, and reps all the *same*.

Take a Week Off

It's time to recover and get to know your sweetheart again. You can still be active so feel free to go biking, swimming, or walking, but stick with lighter activities, and be sure to take it easy. Don't make the same mistake I did: I once filled my rest week with so many strenuous activities that my week "off" was even more intense than my regular workout! So, I had to take a real week off afterward. Remember, the idea is to *rest* your recently taxed muscles. Your body – and your sweetheart – will thank you! Definitely stretch during this period too as this will help "clean out" your muscles and get you ready for your next training cycle.

The Intermediate Workout

It's time to change it up a bit - and time to ramp-up the volume. This routine takes you and your physique to the proverbial "next level". Now's the time to add a few variations to your workout—but don't worry, we're not about to overhaul the entire system. The best and least traumatic way to freshen up your workout is to vary your grips and your stances slightly. Keep the number of days you work out per week, the rest periods between sets, and the weekly percentages the same.

Mondays and Fridays:
- Pull Downs with palms facing your ears: five sets of ten to fifteen reps.
  Or Pull-ups: five sets of ten to fifteen reps.
- Bench Press: five sets of five reps. Move the hands in or out about an inch or so on each side.
- Dips: two sets of ten reps.
- Leg Press: four sets of five reps. Move the feet out an inch or two on each side.
- Sit-ups: four sets of twenty reps. Use ten to fifteen-pound weights.
- Worst Exercise in the World: two times.

Wednesdays:
Keep your Wednesday workout the same. Light all the way.

These changes stress your muscles in different ways and change the dynamic of your workout. You'll want to maintain exceptional technique throughout these exercises. (You know you weren't getting away without a technique reminder!)

The Advanced Workout - The Split Routine
Now you're ready for the *real* good stuff! This workout routine separates the men from the boys. After you've been weight lifting for a while, you're going to want to liberally employ the variations described in the previous chapters. These advanced routines are for the truly dedicated, or fanatics (as my mother calls yours truly), because they take more time and a lot more effort. I've split the workouts up into two sessions to be done on separate days. The lower body workout day consists of leg and abdominal exercises, and the upper body day consists of everything else. While I realize that a convincing argument can made that your abs are really part of your upper body, splitting the workouts up in this way has always worked out pretty well for me - so try it to start out. Upper body workouts are done twice a week: Monday and Friday. Lower body workouts are also done twice a week: Wednesday and Saturday. Also, you will be adjusting your grips and stances once again.

I have found success in going heavy on the bench on Mondays and heavy with the military press on Fridays – always in the same week. I usually lead off with my heaviest exercise first. In addition, I alternate heavy weeks: heavy upper-body one week; heavy lower body the following week. I have found that this is easier both on the body and on the mind.

Upper Body Monday
- Bench Press: five sets of five reps. Note: Week One will be heavy; week two will be light.
- Achievement Pull-ups (palms facing your ears): two times. (See Chapter VII.)
- Seated or Standing Military Press: four sets of five reps. Always light.

Lower Body Wednesday
- Dead Lifts off Blocks: 4 x 5; light to medium weight only. Elevate the bar approx. eight inches off the floor. A Power Rack is ideal for this if you are using an Olympic Bar. If your gym has a Hex-Bar, definitely use that but you'll have to figure out a way to elevate the bar. I have built blocks out of 2 x 12s stacked four high and that works just fine.
- Seated Calf Raises: 4 x 10.
- Worst Exercise in the World: x 2.

Upper Body Friday
- Seated or Standing Military Press: 5 x 5. Note: Week One will be heavy; week two will be light.
- Pull-ups: 8 x 10.
- Bench Press: 6 x 5. Always light.

Lower Body Saturday
- Back Squat: 3 x 5. Note: Week One will be light; week two will be heavy.
- Seated Calf Raises (optional): 2 x 10. Medium weight only.

I've kept the Calf-Raises quick and optional as you just may not feel like it after heavy legs. If you worked your legs right, you will have earned the rest of the day off!

Remember to alternate heavy weeks. Don't lift your heaviest weight every week or you'll burn yourself our very quickly. Remember, this workout routine is an *eight-week* cycle. After those initial eight weeks, you can liberally incorporate variations throughout your routine.

Chapter VIII
Exercises to Avoid

This book wouldn't be complete without a warning label—so here it is. You'll want to avoid these exercises because they are either too technical in nature and doing them improperly can cause injury and at our age, injuries last and last and last, or they put an extraordinary loading on your joints. You can achieve better results safely by doing different exercises entirely—all of which are covered in this book. That being said, you'll want to avoid the following exercises:

- Behind the neck presses
- Pull-downs behind the neck
- Power cleans – very few people know how to do them right and there are so many ways to get injured by doing them wrong.
- Bent-over rows
- Leg extensions
- Any exercise with the term *single arm* in it, i.e. single arm rows, presses, triceps extensions, etc.

Chapter IX
The Younger Generation

This chapter is dedicated to the younger crowd. *Younger* is defined as anyone who does not get up in the morning hunched over and leaning on as many objects as possible for the first few steps. Hangovers don't count. The workouts in this section are designed just for you and are intense. Now, before you go diving right into the sets and reps, you'll need to pay careful and complete attention to Chapter II through Chapter VII. Read the whole book first, and then re-read those sections as they are *critical* to your success in the gym.

One of the fortunate aspects of this stage of your life is that you have a lot going for you, especially, youth and enthusiasm. You also have a few things working against you, namely, youth and enthusiasm. Remember all those mistakes I've referenced throughout the book? Well, I made most of them when I was *young*. If you learn the basics and build from there, you'll extend the period of time in which you'll make gains. If you try to cut corners, even *your* body will eventually show you who's boss (and guess what: it ain't you!).

The One That Got Away
When I was lifting competitively, we would have wannabes rotate in and out of the gym on a regular basis. Oh, they wanted to be lifters—that is, until they saw what weightlifting was really all about: grinding, unglamorous hard work! Enter Nick. Nick had the *perfect* levers, or body proportions, to be a great lifter. Perfect. They were even better than my training partner's and far better than mine! He was already relatively strong too and that actually worked *against* him. The trouble was that he didn't know *how* to lift. The bigger trouble was that he wouldn't allow us to break him down from a technical point of view. He wasn't *"train-able."* He wasn't about to be taught something that he thought he already knew. I was always amazed about how so many lifter-wannabes wouldn't allow nationally-ranked lifter teach them. Quite frankly, one was too many! Eventually, out of frustration, my training partner told him that if he never became national champion, he had no one to blame but himself. You know how long Nick lasted? One week. One frustrating week. During his last training session, he was trying to snatch, and he proceeded to run headlong off the platform with the barbell overhead and straight into the concrete wall. I'm not kidding. He went one way; the bar went the other. No more Olympic lifting for dear Nick. The shame of it was that he could have been *great*, but he let his ego get in his way. Don't let that happen to you. Take the time to learn, learn, learn. The minute you stop critiquing yourself is the minute you're in trouble.

Okay, let's have some fun! I'm going to throw in some very advanced exercises that will tax your athletic skills and help you develop explosive power. We old guys should avoid these as they put extraordinary loading on our aging joints. You young guys can take this and have fun with it.

Clean Pulls from the Medium Blocks
Practically every football coach has advocated *Power Cleans* to their players to help them develop speed and strength. The trouble is that most coaches have no idea how to do them properly, and this lack of knowledge translates into a colossal waste of time and effort. What's even worse is that improper technique actually hinders the athlete trying to do them and does not build power and speed – quite the opposite. I'm going to show you a much better way to build that power and speed - a way which has been proven to bring exceptional results. Before we continue, let's go over a couple of technical points. First, the explosive

power generated in the power clean occurs when the bar *passes* the knees, and second, the power is at its height when the lifter reaches full extension. At that point, the bar reaches the bottom of the lifter's belt. That's it. The rest of the move is nothing more than the momentum of the bar reaching the lifter's shoulders, and that is where just about everyone gets into trouble. They start pulling with the arms before the bar reaches the belt, which causes the back to hunch over, slowing down the lift and defeating the entire purpose of the lift. So, we're going to cut out the *clean* part of the lift and just focus on the *pull* part. By the way, my training partner hardly ever did power cleans, and yet he clean and jerked 457 pounds! How? He mastered the clean *pull*, which I am going to teach you now. Insignificant Historical Note: even I out power-cleaned him, and I really wasn't any good at it. How much did I do? 330 pounds.

First, you'll need to make two wooden blocks: nail six two-by-twelves on top of each other. Tack a rubber mat on top of each one because the wood will really get beat up if you don't. These are called "The Medium Blocks." If you can set the power rack up so that the bar is at knee height at the start of the lift, that's just as good. One last point: this lift is a very technical one, and it is the most difficult part of the Olympic lifts to master. Once you get it though, you will be amazed at how this builds power and strength!

Next, you'll need straps to help you maintain your grip on the bar. You can either buy them or use my method, which is to cut two twenty-inch sections from an old belt and use them as follows: wrap them around your wrist and hold the two ends with your thumb and forefinger. Holding the ends together, wrap them under the bar and slide your hand on top of them. This will give you a very secure grip.

The Start
Place the bar on the blocks and get your knees right up to the bar. Your legs should be straight and about shoulder-width apart, and your toes should be underneath the bar. Point your toes outward, turn your elbows outward, curl your hands inward, push your shoulders down, arch your back, and push your stomach out hard against the belt. These instructions are important keys, and at this point, you have not yet bent over to grasp the bar. As you lean over, maintain all of the above positioning, and point your knees in the direction of your toes. Do not allow the bar to roll out and away from you. This is imperative! Grab the bar, placing your hands a little wider than shoulder-width apart, and lower your hips until your shoulders are slightly ahead of the bar. Your weight should be on your heels. This stance is the *starting* position.

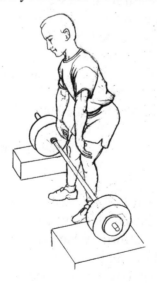

Personal Story

When I first started learning all of this positioning, I was thinking all the things that you are probably thinking right now: "This *can't* be right! I feel like a contortionist!" My training partner (you know - the one who made the Olympic Team) pulled me aside one evening and told me one very important thing: "Weight lifting is not comfortable." Man, was he right! It's not comfortable, especially at first. However, once you get the hang of it, it will be. Be patient and allow yourself the time to learn.

The Pull

Now that you are in the proper position, you are ready for the *pull* part of the lift. *Steadily* push upward with your legs, keeping your back tight and at roughly the same angle as your starting position. Do not jerk the bar from the blocks as it will throw off your positioning and may cause your back to bend forward (called *breaking*). When the bar reaches the *top* of your thighs, shift your weight from your heels to your toes while keeping your shoulders up (not back). This move is known as the infamous *double-knee bend* or *scoop*. Do not allow your shoulders to fade backwards. If you've been doing deadlifts, this part will be the hardest to correct. Remember: shoulders up, not back! The bar should come in contact with your upper thighs, very close to your hips. The next move is easy: just jump straight up. Straighten your legs and shrug your shoulders, and keep those arms absolutely *straight*! The bar should hit the bottom of your belt if you're doing it right. The audible *click* will be your sign that you've don't the pull correctly. Note: your arms are completely *useless* during the pull. Useless. They do not supply *any* power to the pull, and if you bend them prematurely, they only serve to slow you down. When I first started weight lifting, I was told to think of them as ropes - something that is merely holding onto the bar. You'd be well-advised to think of them the same way. During an actual squat clean, your arms are used to pull you under the weight. That's right: they pull *you* down; they do not pull the weight up! Most of the power is supplied by your thighs and hips during the pull, which lasts until the lifter's legs are fully extended and his shoulders are shrugged. For our purposes, that's where the move stops. When you do this right, the bar will accelerate at the top of the pull, right after the double-knee bend. Now you're developing both strength and speed!

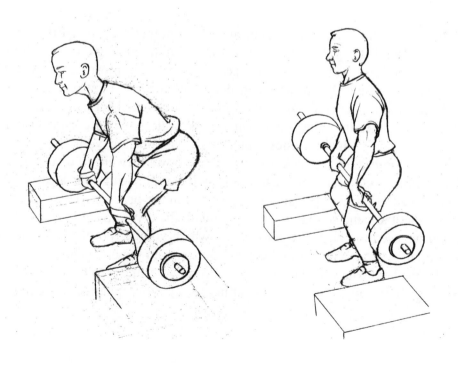

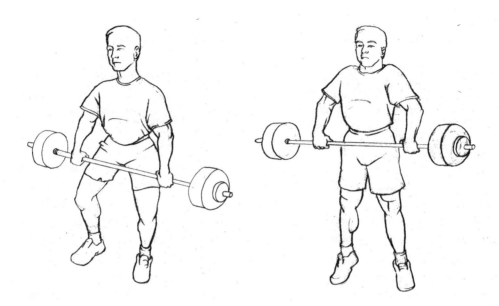

Now do you see why I started out with a broomstick? I advise you to do the same. You should be able to learn this properly in a couple of months. Yes, months. Have patience, grasshopper.

At this point, you may be wondering, "Why on earth should I learn this stuff? I'm never going to be a competitive lifter." True that, whipper-snapper. But here's why: in just about every sport (e.g. baseball, softball, golf, tennis, and football), hip strength and explosive power are the keys to success. Watch a major league player swing the bat: he "unwinds" from his feet to his shoulders with his hips supplying most of the power. Clean pulls help you develop dynamic power and speed that carries over into these other sports. The simple fact is that learning these lifts will help you perform better in your sport of choice.

Overheads

These are known as *push jerks* in weightlifter lingo, and it is another technical lift, but it's not nearly as difficult as the clean pull. This lift is yet another great way to build explosive power and strength. This is the *jerk* part of the clean-and-jerk, and it is often misapplied because most people don't understand the mechanics of the lift. Guess what? We're about to change that too! First and foremost, eliminate the thought that this is a lift in which you simply drive the weight overhead. That's only half the story; the other half is where real athleticism comes into play – and which most athletes never even considered. We'll get to that a bit later. Let's first start with the basics: grasp the bar, placing your hands slightly wider than shoulder-width apart. Take the bar off the rack, extend your elbows forward like you do in the front squat, and make sure the bar is resting on your clavicles. Stand bolt upright with your legs slightly bent. Take a sharp two-inch dip and drive the weight up, rising on your toes in the process. The idea of a short but sharp dip is to *stop* the bar, getting it to bend so that it assists you with the drive upward. I repeat: *stop* the bar! Do not do a *soft* dip, which we used to call that a *flat tire*, in which you get no bounce whatsoever. I've seen countless lifters take a dip of six to ten inches and get no bounce from the bar. The mechanics behind the dip is sort of like judo: make the bar (your opponent) work for you by getting it to bend and throw itself upward. Be sure to make your dip short and sharp. (I'm repeating myself to emphasize my point, not because I'm old.)

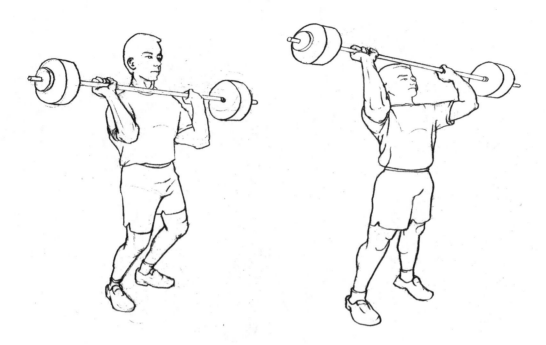

The next part of the lift is absolutely critical for you to understand and then to execute. This part is where most lifters miss the point. Once the drive has been made, you can supply *no more power* to the bar. Zero, zip, nada. So, *push yourself underneath the bar* by squatting under it. Yes, push yourself *down*, not the weight up. Notice a theme here? Your arms do *very little* as far as supplying power to these dynamic moves. You will meet the bar at its highest point, and of course, the highest point will be determined by how much weight you are lifting. Generally, you drive the bar no higher than the top of your forehead on the heavier lifts. More experienced lifters will be able to jump their feet apart to catch the weight once the drive has been made. Jumping the feet apart is much easier if you rise on your toes during the drive upwards, which makes the move more natural. So, do a short, sharp two-inch dip followed by a drive up on the toes. Push yourself underneath the bar to meet it at its highest point.

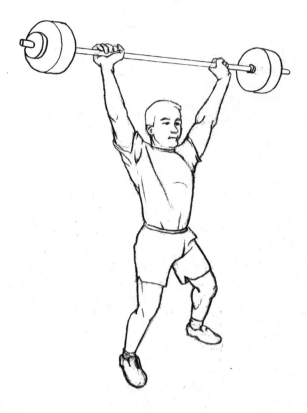

Did I mention that the *pull* and the *overhead* will build your entire back, trapezius, arm, and shoulder muscles all at the same time? As I mentioned before, I believe in training your muscles in groups.

Basic Training

If you've never cast a shadow across a barbell before, then your initial workout is going to be pretty much the same as the "Beginner Workout" outlined in Chapter V. You'll want to stick with this routine for the same twelve-week timeframe. This routine will help you build a base and avoid the soreness that accompanies a more intense workout. My objective is to keep you moving forward as opposed to having you think, "What the heck have I gotten myself into?" Once you've done this twelve-week session, you can move on to the intermediate workout below.

The Intermediate Workout

For you younger folks, we're ratcheting up the intensity level and helping you build a broader base. Do this twice a week.

- Pull Downs, palms facing your ears: six sets of ten to fifteen reps.
  Or Pull-ups: six sets of ten to fifteen reps.
- Bench Press: five sets of five reps. Move the hands in or out about an inch or so on each side.
- Dips: three sets of ten reps.
- Seated Alternate Press: three sets of ten reps.
- Leg Press: four sets of five reps. Move the feet out an inch or two on each side.
- Good Mornings: three sets of ten reps.
- Sit-ups: five sets of twenty reps. Use ten to fifteen pounds.

- Worst Exercise in the World: two times.

Be sure to move the hands and feet out a bit in order to keep the exercises fresh. Also, cut the rest period to two to three minutes between sets. Finally, be sure to take that week off at the end of this cycle!

The Advanced Workout - The Split Routine

Now it's time to incorporate speed, power, and body building into one nice, neat little package! Keep in mind that you will need to take a week off between cycles. This rest week is *critical* as you will definitely need and welcome the rest. Similar to the advanced routines in Chapter V, these workouts are *split routines*, meaning that the routines are divided into two days: you'll work out your upper body on one day and your lower body on another. Upper-body days are Monday and Friday; lower-body day is Saturday with Wednesday being a "combination" day incorporating both upper-body and lower-body exercises. Start out with three-minute rest periods between sets. After six weeks, reduce your rest periods to two minutes.

Monday
- Achievement Pull-ups, palms facing your ears: two times. (See Chapter VII.)
- Inclined Bench Press: five sets of five reps.
- Dumbbell Bench Press: three sets of eight to twelve reps.
- Worst Exercise in the World: three times.
- Sit-ups: five sets of twenty reps. For heavy weeks, add twenty-five to fifty pounds. Also, make sure you perform the repetitions slowly.

Alternate heavy- and light-weight weeks.

Wednesday
- Push Jerks: five sets of three reps. Light to moderate weight.
- Clean Pulls: five sets of three reps. After six weeks, add three sets. Moderate weight.
- Good Mornings: four sets of five reps. For heavy weeks, use moderate to heavy weight.
- Leg Press: four sets of ten reps. Light to moderate weight.
- Ab Work: The Eight-minute Drill. (See Chapter VII.)

Friday
- Bench Press: eight sets of five reps. Drop the weight by twenty percent and add an extra rep for the last three sets. Alternate heavy- and light-weight weeks.
- Pull Ups, palms facing your ears: four sets of fifteen reps.
- Pull-Ups, palms facing you: four sets of ten to fifteen reps.
- Worst Exercise in the World: two times.
- Ab Work: Achievement Leg Lifts. (Do not use any weight.)

Saturday
- Back Squats: four sets of five reps.
- Clean Pulls: five sets of three reps. After six weeks, add three sets.

Alternate heavy and light weeks.

Chapter X
The Final Chapter

We all know that teaching an old dog new tricks is a bit of a challenge. Staying out of competitive weightlifting has been equally challenging for me as I've always longed to get back on the platform. Over the years, however, my joints would revolt every time I dabbled in Olympic lifting (yes, my body proved to be smarter that I am—again!). So, after a while, even I figured out that, for me, Olympic weightlifting was now part of the good old days.

Then, quite by accident, I found myself traveling headlong for another rendezvous with the platform. I felt as though I just took one baby step without really looking and was suddenly thrust onto another roller coaster ride! It started out innocently enough: I was bored with my leg workout. Yes, yours truly can get bored with lifting too. For years, I was content (I thought) to leg press my life away—and, yes, I did all the variations I told you about too—but my leg workouts were becoming, well, boring. There are only so many ways that you can leg press. For years, I was reluctant to start squatting again because of my on-again-off-again banged up left knee. One day, I gave myself a devastatingly motivational talking-to: "The hell with it. Just do it, you idiot." Well, well… With that, I started squatting again.

After a few workouts, I got the hang of it again and was pleasantly surprised at my progress. I went from 185 to 225 pounds for reps pretty comfortably. Now, of course, I could *never* be satisfied squatting light weights. I had to see how far I could go. I adjusted my leg press stance to a wider one, which shifted the stress of the weights more to my hips and would help me squat a higher weight (these are some of the tricks of the trade that you learn over the years). Leg pressing suddenly became an *assist exercise* and squatting became my main exercise. I smirked at my cleverness, and away went the leg workout boredom-factor. Then, in a move that surprised absolutely nobody, I entered a squat contest. I think my wife's reaction was "I hope you know what you're doing." By that time, it didn't really matter because my destiny was set: I was going to compete again!

Naturally, I was under a bit of time pressure as the meet was only eight weeks away! So, instead of just having fun with it, I immediately intensified my training, and almost just as immediately, I tweaked my left knee again. (Will I ever learn?) While the injury slowed me down a bit, it wasn't going to stop this old dog. I moderated my training and aggressively rehabbed my knee. I did another smart thing too. Remember how I told you to keep a notebook, a record of your weights, sets, and reps? Well, I took it one step further: I set goals that I would hit the day of the meet. If you are determined to get stronger, making goals is a *great* way to stay on track. For some reason, setting goals really focuses your mind, and your body just responds. No, it's not magic, but it's pretty close!

So, I took a deep breath, focused on my target weights and started to enjoy my training again. Ten days before the meet, I hit 315 pounds for a triple (three reps), which was actually more than I thought I'd do considering my knee-tweakage of a few weeks before. I was feeling pretty confident.

The day of my competition arrived, and I began to wonder what the heck I was doing there. "You should be home cutting the grass, feeding the turtles—anything but going to this stupid meet! What on earth is wrong with you?" However, I got over my pre-meet jitters pretty quickly and started to enjoy the day. The whole experience was made extra- special because not only were my wife and my twenty-something daughter there but also a good friend and weightlifter from my Olympic lifting days was going to help me through the day! I couldn't have been more excited! In addition, I was going to use my thirty-two-year-old weightlifting shoes, my thirty-two-year-old weightlifting belt and my thirty-two-year-old weightlifting uniform on my fifty-plus-year-old body! What fun!

I knew I was in for a different-kind-of-interesting day when the weigh-in was conducted by a female gym member. For what should be obvious reasons, weigh-ins are normally - the operative term here is "normally" - conducted while in your birthday-suit in the men's locker room and are supervised by the male referees. This day, however, the competitors weighed-in fully clothed, and everyone else seemed to feel that this was pretty, well, normal. (Cue the Twilight Zone music). The weigh-in wouldn't be the last oddity of the day. Later, when I asked where I could stretch because, as a former Olympic-style lifter, I knew the benefit of flexibility, I got the following shrug-of-the-shoulders answer: "This is power-lifting. We don't stretch." (Cue the Twilight Zone music again, please.) In any event, I did manage to find a closet-sized room where I stretched out, and I didn't have to worry about sharing!

The meet was about to start, and being a nervous Nellie, I warmed up a bit too soon. But it really didn't matter a whole lot because I was pretty pumped mentally. Lifters have three attempts at each lift, and I figured I'd start out with a safe weight of 315 pounds. I made it smoothly enough and, when I heard the announcer say something like "Wow, that was really easy", I figured I was in for a good day! I must say that it was a curious feeling to hear a "Go, Dad!" each time I stepped up to the bar! My next attempt was 330 pounds, and I received two reds (two red lights means the lift is no good) for not going deep enough in the squat. Remember, the tops of your thighs must be parallel to the floor. My friend was pretty agitated about the call. No, he didn't make a scene; he just groused about it until he felt better. (Funny Note: we met at another meet a few years later, and he was still bitching about it!) It felt great to have his unconditional support! Nevertheless, I decided to move up to my target weight of the day for my final attempt: 340 pounds. By the way, increasing your weight after missing a lighter one is usually ill-advised. But whoever said I was conventional?

I was getting pretty tired by then as the meet seemed to go on forever. I had to stay warm by doing light squats over and over. Finally, I was called for my last attempt. I approached the bar (yes, to another "Go, Dad!"), got set, and took the bar off the rack. Quite frankly, it felt really heavy—like the weight of the world. The ref took his sweet time giving me the signal to "Squat!"—and away I went. Down into the bottom, which felt miles away. After I dropped for what seemed like an eternity, my instincts took over, I felt my glutes tighten in the bottom, and I started coming out of the abyss. I struggled half-way up, forcing my knees out and my hips in (remember that trick?), and to the cheering of the crowd, I made it successfully! Three whites! I was an exhausted, happy camper.

Walking off the platform, I hugged and thanked my dear friend. We sat and chatted for a while, but eventually, we had to say good-bye. I sat with my wife and daughter for a bit, taking in the whole surreal scene. Finally, I mustered the energy to go to the locker room to clean up. I ran into one of the refs, who was about my age and a former Olympic-style lifter as well, and he warmly congratulated me for my last attempt. I dressed in my street clothes, gathered my things, and sat for a few minutes pondering about my day, my family, and my friend. Even though 340 pounds for one rep is a long way from 500 pounds for five reps, I'm also a long way from twenty-five years old! I got up, looked in the mirror, and thought, "Not bad for an old man!"

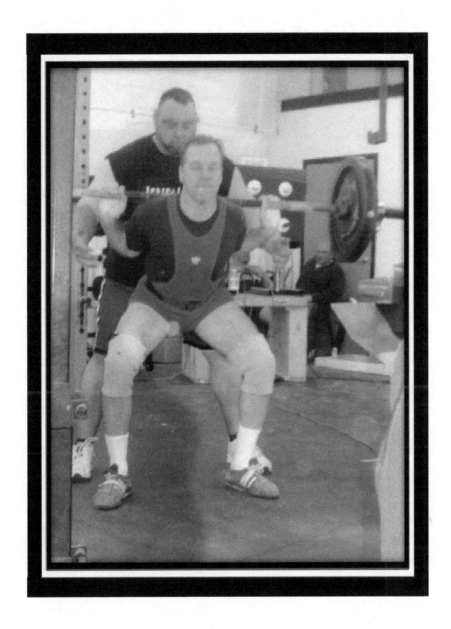

CPSIA information can be obtained
at www.ICGtesting.com
Printed in the USA
BVHW08s0846210818
524961BV00008B/79/P